Sirt Diet Snacks and Desserts

By

Lola Matten

Sirt Diet Snacks and Desserts

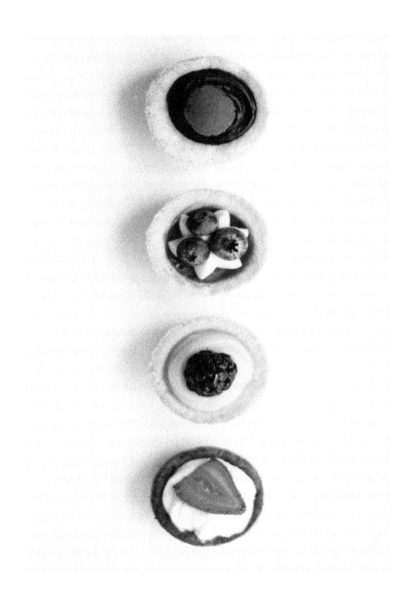

Sirt Diet Snacks and Desserts

© Copyright 2021 by Lola Matten

fashion deemed liable for any hardship or damages that may befall them after undertaking information described herein.

Additionally, the information in the following pages is intended only for informational purposes and should thus be thought of as universal. As befitting its nature, it is presented without assurance regarding its prolonged validity or interim quality. Trademarks that are mentioned are done without written consent and can in no way be considered an endorsement from the trademark holder.

Table of Contents

6

Sirt Diet Snacks and Desserts

Baby Spinach Snack

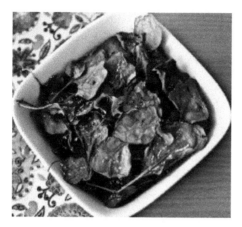

Preparation time: 10 minutes

Cooking time: 10 minutes

Servings: 1

Ingredients:

2 cups baby spinach, washed

A pinch of black pepper

½ tablespoon olive oil

½ teaspoon garlic powder

Directions:

Spread the baby spinach on a lined baking sheet, add oil, black pepper and garlic powder, toss a bit.

Bake at 350 degrees F for 10 minutes, divide into bowls and serve as a snack.

Enjoy!

Nutrition:

Calories: 125

Fat: 4 g

Fiber: 1 g

Carbohydrates: 4 g

Protein: 2 g

Sesame Dip

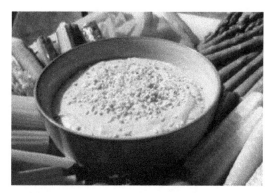

Preparation time: 10 minutes

Cooking time: 0 minutes

Servings: 1

Ingredients:

1 cup sesame seed paste, pure

Black pepper to the taste

1 cup veggie stock

½ cup lemon juice

½ teaspoon cumin, ground

3 garlic cloves, chopped

Directions:

In your food processor, mix the sesame paste with black pepper, stock, lemon juice, cumin and garlic.

Pulse very well, divide into bowls and serve as a party dip.

Enjoy!

Nutrition:

Calories: 120

Fat: 12 g

Fiber: 2 g

Carbohydrates: 7 g

Protein: 4 g

Rosemary Squash Dip

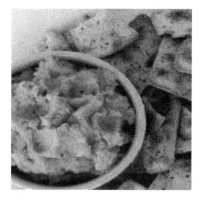

Preparation time: 10 minutes

Cooking time: 40 minutes

Servings: 1

Ingredients:

1 cup butternut squash, peeled and cubed

1 tablespoon water

Cooking spray

2 tablespoons coconut milk

2 teaspoons rosemary, dried

Black pepper to the taste

Directions:

Spread squash cubes on a lined baking sheet, spray some cooking oil, introduce in the oven, bake at 365 degrees F for 40 minutes.

Transfer to your blender, add water, milk, rosemary and black pepper, pulse well, divide into small bowls and serve.

Enjoy!

Nutrition:

Calories: 182

Fat: 5 g

Fiber: 7 g

Carbohydrates: 12 g

Protein: 5 g

Bean Spread

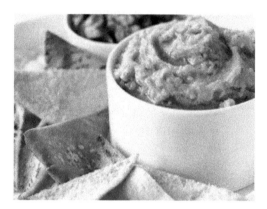

Preparation time: 10 minutes

Cooking time: 6 hours

Servings: 1

Ingredients:

1 cup white beans, dried

1 teaspoon apple cider vinegar

1 cup veggie stock

1 tablespoon water

Directions:

In your slow cooker, mix beans with stock, stir, cover, cook on Low for 6 hours.

Drain and transfer to your food processor, add vinegar and water, pulse well, divide into bowls and serve.

Enjoy!

Nutrition:

Calories: 181

Fat: 6 g

Fiber: 5 g

Carbohydrates: 9 g

Protein: 7 g

Corn Spread

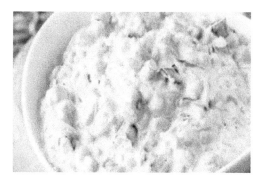

Preparation time: 10 minutes

Cooking time: 10 minutes

Servings: 1

Ingredients:

30 ounces canned corn, drained

2 green onions, chopped

½ cup coconut cream

1 jalapeno, chopped

½ teaspoon chili powder

Directions:

In a small pan, combine the corn with green onions, jalapeno and chili powder, stir, and bring to a simmer.

Cook over medium heat for 10 minutes, leave aside to cool down, add coconut cream, stir well, divide into small bowls and serve as a spread.

Enjoy!

Nutrition:

Calories: 192

Fat: 5

Fiber 10

Carbohydrates: 11 g

Protein: 8 g

Mushroom Dip

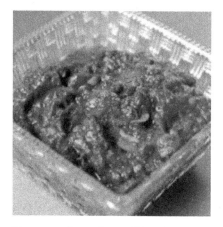

Preparation time: 10 minutes

Cooking time: 20 minutes

Servings: 1

Ingredients:

1 cup yellow onion, chopped

3 garlic cloves, minced

1 pound mushrooms, chopped

28 ounces tomato sauce, no-salt-added

Black pepper to the taste

Directions:

Put the onion in a pot, add garlic, mushrooms, black pepper and tomato sauce, and stir.

Cook over medium heat for 20 minutes, leave aside to cool down, divide into small bowls and serve.

Enjoy!

Nutrition:

Calories 215

Fat: 4 g

Fiber: 7 g

Carbohydrates: 3 g

Protein: 7 g

Salsa Bean Dip

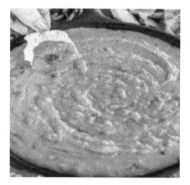

Preparation time: 10 minutes

Cooking time: 20 minutes

Servings: 1

Ingredients:

½ cup salsa

2 cups canned white beans, no-salt-added, drained and rinsed

1 cup low-fat cheddar, shredded

2 tablespoons green onions, chopped

Directions:

In a small pot, combine the beans with the green onions and salsa, stir, bring to a simmer over medium heat, and cook for 20 minutes Add cheese, stir until it melts, and take off heat, leave aside to cool down, divide into bowls and serve.

Enjoy!

Nutrition:

Calories: 212

Fat: 5 g

Fiber: 6 g

Carbohydrates: 10 g

Protein: 8 g

Mung Beans Snack Salad

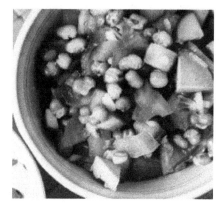

Preparation time: 10 minutes

Cooking time: 0 minutes

Servings: 1

Ingredients:

2 cups tomatoes, chopped

2 cups cucumber, chopped

3 cups mixed greens

2 cups mung beans, sprouted

2 cups clover sprouts

For the salad dressing:

1 tablespoon cumin, ground

1 cup dill, chopped

4 tablespoons lemon juice

1 avocado, pitted, peeled and roughly chopped

1 cucumber, roughly chopped

Directions:

In a salad bowl, mix tomatoes with 2 cups cucumber, greens, clover and mung sprout.

In your blender, mix cumin with dill, lemon juice, 1 cucumber and avocado, blend really well, add this to your salad, toss well and serve as a snack

Enjoy!

Nutrition:

Calories: 120

Fat: 0 g

Fiber: 2 g

Carbohydrates: 1 g

Protein: 6 g

Greek Party Dip

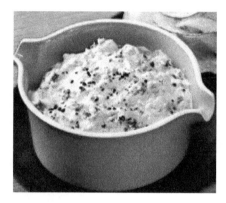

Preparation time: 10 minutes

Cooking time: 0 minutes

Servings: 1

Ingredients:

½ cup coconut cream

1 cup fat-free Greek yogurt

2 teaspoons dill, dried

2 teaspoons thyme, dried

1 teaspoon sweet paprika

2 teaspoons no-salt-added sun-dried tomatoes, chopped

2 teaspoons parsley, chopped

2 teaspoons chives, chopped

Black pepper to the taste

Directions:

In a bowl, mix cream with yogurt, dill with thyme, paprika, tomatoes, parsley, chives and pepper, stir well.

Divide into smaller bowls and serve as a dip.

Enjoy!

Nutrition:

Calories: 100

Fat: 1 g

Fiber: 4 g

Carbohydrates: 8 g

Protein: 3 g

Zucchini Bowls

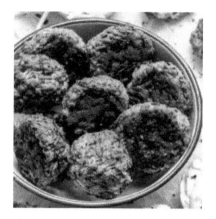

Preparation time: 10 minutes

Cooking time: 20 minutes

Servings: 12

Ingredients:

Cooking spray

½ cup dill, chopped

1 egg

½ cup whole wheat flour

Black pepper to the taste

1 yellow onion, chopped

2 garlic cloves, minced

3 zucchinis, grated

Directions:

In a bowl, mix zucchinis with garlic, onion, flour, pepper, egg and dill, stir well, shape small bowls out of this mix.

Arrange them on a lined baking sheet; grease them with some cooking spray.

Bake at 400 degrees F for 20 minutes, flipping them halfway, divide them into bowls and serve as a snack.

Enjoy!

Nutrition:

Calories: 120

Fat: 1 g

Fiber: 4 g

Carbohydrates: 12 g

Protein: 6 g

Baking Powder Biscuits

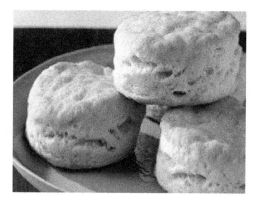

Preparation time: 10 minutes

Cooking time: 10 minutes

Servings: 1 2

Ingredients:

1 egg white

1 c. white whole-wheat flour

4 tbsp. of Non-hydrogenated vegetable shortening

1 tbsp. sugar

2/3 c. low-fat milk

1 c. unbleached all-purpose flour

4 tsps. Sodium-free baking powder

Directions:

Preheat oven to 450°F. Take out a baking sheet and set aside.

Place the flour, sugar, and baking powder into a mixing bowl and whisk well to combine.

Cut the shortening into the mixture using your fingers, and work until it resembles coarse crumbs. Add the egg white and milk and stir to combine.

Turn the dough out onto a lightly floured surface and knead 1 minute. Roll dough to ¾ inch thickness and cut into 12 rounds.

Place rounds on the baking sheet. Place baking sheet on middle rack in oven and bake 10 minutes.

Remove baking sheet and place biscuits on a wire rack to cool.

Nutrition:

Calories: 118

Fat: 4 g

Carbohydrates: 16 g

Protein: 3 g

Sugars: 0.2 g

Sodium: 294 mg

Vegan Rice Pudding

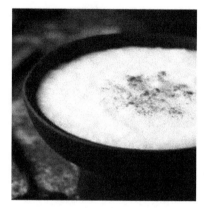

Preparation time: 5 minutes

Cooking time: 20 minutes

Servings: 8

Ingredients:

½ tsp. ground cinnamon

1 c. rinsed basmati

1/8 tsp. ground cardamom

¼ c. sugar

1/8 tsp. pure almond extract

1 quart vanilla nondairy milk

1 tsp. pure vanilla extract

Directions:

Measure all of the ingredients into a saucepan and stir well to combine. Bring to a boil over medium-high heat.

Once boiling, reduce heat to low and simmer, stirring very frequently, about 15–20 minutes.

Remove from heat and cool. Serve sprinkled with additional ground cinnamon if desired.

Nutrition:

Calories: 148

Fat: 2 g

Carbohydrates: 26 g

Protein: 4 g

Sugars: 35 g

Sodium: 150 mg

Orange and Carrots

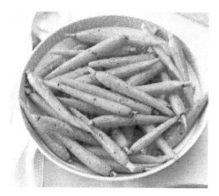

Preparation time: 5 minutes

Cooking time: 25 minutes

Servings: 1

Ingredients:

1 pound carrots, peeled and roughly sliced

1 yellow onion, chopped

1 tablespoon olive oil

Zest of 1 orange, grated

Juice of 1 orange

1 orange, peeled and cut into segments

1 tablespoon rosemary, chopped

A pinch of salt and black pepper

Directions:

Heat up a pan with the oil over medium-high heat.

Add the onion and sauté for 5 minutes.

Add the carrots, the orange zest and the other ingredients.

Cook over medium heat for 20 minutes more, divide between plates and serve.

Nutrition:

Calories: 140

Fat: 3.9 g

Fiber: 5 g

Carbohydrates: 26.1 g

Protein: 2.1 g

Baked Broccoli and Pine Nuts

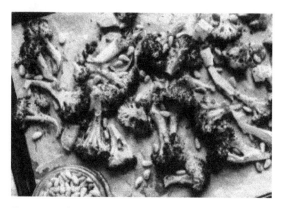

Preparation time: 10 minutes

Cooking time: 30 minutes

Servings: 1

Ingredients:

2 tablespoons olive oil

1 pound broccoli florets

1 tablespoon garlic, minced

1 tablespoon pine nuts, toasted

1 tablespoon lemon juice

2 teaspoons mustard

A pinch of salt and black pepper

Directions:

In a roasting pan, combine the broccoli with the oil, the garlic and the other ingredients, toss and bake at 380 degrees F for 30 minutes. Divide everything between plates and serve as snack.

Nutrition:

Calories: 220

Fat: 6 g

Fiber: 2 g

Carbohydrates: 7 g

Protein: 6 g

Turmeric Carrots

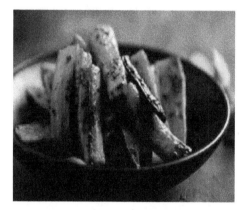

Preparation time: 10 minutes

Cooking time: 40 minutes

Servings: 1

Ingredients:

1 pound baby carrots, peeled

1 tablespoon olive oil

2 spring onions, chopped

2 tablespoons balsamic vinegar

2 garlic cloves, minced

1 teaspoon turmeric powder

1 tablespoon chives, chopped

¼ teaspoon cayenne pepper

A pinch of salt and black pepper

Directions:

Spread the carrots on a baking sheet lined with parchment paper, add the oil, the spring onions and the other ingredients, toss and bake at 380 degrees F for 40 minutes.

Divide the carrots between plates and serve.

Nutrition:

Calories: 79

Fat: 3.8 g

Fiber: 3.7 g

Carbohydrates: 10.9 g

Protein: 1 g

Hawaii Salad

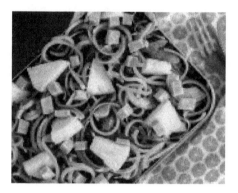

Preparation time: 10 minutes

Cooking time: 15 minutes

Servings: 1

Ingredients:

1 hand Arugula

1 / 2 pieces Red onion

1 piece winter carrot

2 pieces Pineapple slices

80 g Diced ham

1 pinch Salt

1 pinch Black pepper

Directions:

Cut the red onion into thin half rings.

Remove the peel and hard core from the pineapple and cut the pulp into thin pieces.

Clean the carrot and use a spiralizer to make strings.

Mix rocket and carrot in a bowl. Spread this over a plate.

Spread the red onion, pineapple and diced ham over the rocket.

Drizzle olive oil and balsamic vinegar on the salad to your taste.

Season it with salt and pepper.

Nutrition:

Calories: 150

Total Fat: 2.8 g

Cholesterol: 2 mg

Sodium: 42 mg

Potassium: 172 mg

Carbohydrates: 23 g

Protein: 2 g

Fresh Salad with Orange Dressing

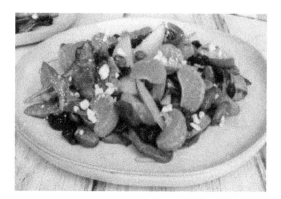

Preparation time: 10 minutes

Cooking time: 15 minutes

Servings: 1

Ingredients:

1 / 2 fruit Salad

1 piece yellow bell pepper

1 piece Red pepper

100 g Carrot (grated)

1 hand Almonds

Dressing:

4 tablespoon Olive oil

110 ml Orange juice (fresh)

1 tablespoon Apple cider vinegar

Directions:

Clean the peppers and cut them into long thin strips.

Tear off the lettuce leaves and cut them into smaller pieces.

Mix the salad with the peppers and the carrots processed in a bowl.

Roughly chop the almonds and sprinkle over the salad.

Mix all the ingredients for the dressing in a bowl.

Pour the dressing over the salad just before serving.

Nutrition:

Calories: 46.6

Total Fat: 0.1 g

Sodium: 230.8 mg

Potassium: 35.6 mg

Total Carbohydrates: 5.6 g

Protein: 0.7 g

Sweet Potato Hash Brown

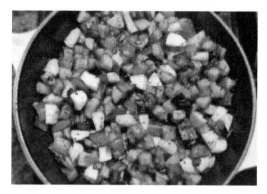

Preparation time: 5 minutes

Cooking time: 15 minutes

Servings: 2

Ingredients:

1 pinch Celtic sea salt

1 tablespoon Coconut oil

2 pieces Sweet potato

2 pieces Red onion

2 teaspoons Balsamic vinegar

1 piece Apple

125 g lean bacon strips

Directions:

Clean the red onions and cut them into half rings.

Heat a pan with a little coconut oil over medium heat. Fry the onion until it's almost done.

Add the balsamic vinegar and a pinch of salt and cook until the balsamic vinegar has boiled down. Put aside.

Peel the sweet potatoes and cut them into approx. 1.5 cm cubes.

Heat the coconut oil in a pan and fry the sweet potato cubes for 10 minutes.

Add the bacon strips for the last 2 minutes and fry them until you're done.

Cut the apple into cubes and add to the sweet potato cubes. Let it roast for a few minutes.

Then add the red onion and stir well.

Spread the sweet potato hash browns on 2 plates.

Nutrition:

Calories: 101

Total Fat: 7 g

Sodium: 5 mg

Potassium: 97 mg

Carbohydrates: 9 g

Protein: 0.8 g

Herby French Fries with Herbs and Avocado Dip

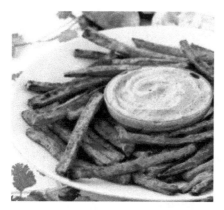

Preparation time: 15 minutes

Cooking time: 35 minutes

Servings: 1

Ingredient:

For the Fries:

1 / 2 pieces Celery

150 g Sweet potato

1 teaspoon dried oregano

1 / 2 teaspoon Dried basil

1 / 2 teaspoon Celtic sea salt

1 teaspoon Black pepper

1 1/2 tablespoon Coconut oil (melted)

Baking paper sheet

For the avocado dip:

1 piece Avocado

4 tablespoons Olive oil

1 tablespoon Mustard

1 teaspoon Apple cider vinegar

1 tablespoon Honey

2 cloves Garlic (pressed)

1 teaspoon dried oregano

Directions:

Preheat the oven to 205 ° C.

Peel the celery and sweet potatoes.

Cut the celery and sweet potatoes into (thin) French fries.

Place the French fries in a large bowl and mix with the coconut oil and herbs.

Shake the bowl a few times so that the fries are covered with a layer of the oil and herb mixture.

Place the chips in a layer on a baking sheet lined with baking paper or on a grill rack.

47

Bake for 25-35 minutes (turn over after half the time) until they have a nice golden brown color and are crispy.

For the avocado dip:

Puree all ingredients evenly with a hand blender or blender.

Nutrition:

Calories: 459

Total Fat: 27 g

Total Carbohydrates: 50 g

Protein: 4 g

Spiced Burger

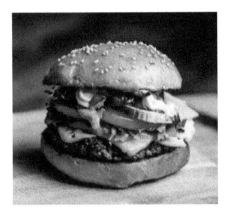

Preparation time: 20 minutes

Cooking time: 30 minutes

Serving: 1

Ingredients:

Ground beef 250 g

1 clove Garlic

1 teaspoon dried oregano

1 teaspoon Paprika powder

1 / 2 tsp. Caraway ground

Ingredients toppings:

4 pieces Mushrooms

1 piece Little Gem

49

1/4 pieces Zucchini

1/2 pieces Red onion

1 piece Tomato

Directions:

Squeeze the clove of garlic.

Mix all the ingredients for the burgers in a bowl. Divide the mixture into two halves and crush the halves into hamburgers.

Place the burgers on a plate and put in the fridge for a while.

Cut the zucchini diagonally into 1 cm slices.

Cut the red onion into half rings. Cut the tomato into thin slices and cut the leaves of the Little Gem salad.

Grill the hamburgers on the grill until they're done.

Place the mushrooms next to the burgers and grill on both sides until cooked but firm.

Place the zucchini slices next to it and grill briefly.

Now it's time to build the burger: Place 2 mushrooms on a plate then stack the lettuce, a few slices of zucchini and tomatoes. Then put the burger on top and finally add the red onion.

Nutrition:

Calories: 158

Fat: 8 g

Total Carbohydrates: 17 g

Protein: 3 g

Ganache Squares

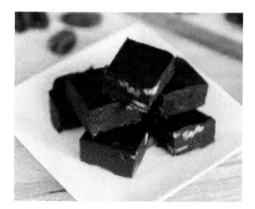

Preparation time: 15 minutes

Cooking time: 2 hours and 20 minutes

Servings: 10

Ingredients:

250 ml Coconut milk (can)

1 1/2 tablespoon Coconut oil

100 g Honey

1/2 teaspoon Vanilla extract

350 g pure chocolate (70% cocoa)

1 pinch Salt

2 hands Pecans

Directions:

Place the coconut milk in a saucepan and heat for 5 minutes over medium heat.

Add the vanilla extract, coconut oil and honey and cook for 15 minutes. Add a pinch of salt and stir well.

Break the chocolate into a bowl and pour the hot coconut milk over it. Keep stirring until all of the chocolate has dissolved in the coconut milk.

In the meantime, roughly chop the pecans. Heat a pan without oil and roast the pecans.

Stir the pecans through the ganache.

Let the ganache cool to room temperature. (You may be able to speed this up by placing the bowl in a bowl of cold water.)

Line a baking tin with a sheet of parchment paper. Pour the cooled ganache into it.

Place the ganache in the refrigerator for 2 hours to allow it to harden. When the ganache has hardened, you can take it out of the mold and cut it into the desired shape.

Nutrition:

Calories: 141

Fat: 11 g

Carbohydrates: 9 g

Protein: 1 g

Date Candy

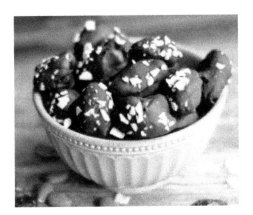

Preparation time: 20 minutes

Cooking time: 3 – 4 hours

Servings: 10

Ingredients:

10 pieces Medjool dates

1 hand Almonds

100 g pure chocolate (70% cocoa)

2 1/2 tablespoon Grated coconut

Directions:

Melt chocolate in a water bath.

Roughly chop the almonds.

In the meantime, cut the dates lengthways and take out the core.

Fill the resulting cavity with the roughly chopped almonds and close the dates again.

Place the dates on a sheet of parchment paper and pour the melted chocolate over each date.

Sprinkle the grated coconut over the chocolate dates.

Place the dates in the fridge so the chocolate can harden.

Nutrition:

100% joy!

Paleo Bars with Dates and Nuts

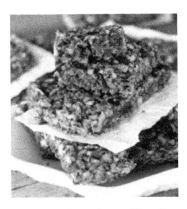

Preparation time: 10 minutes

Cooking time: 15 minutes

Servings: 16

Ingredients:

180 g Dates

60 g Almonds

60 g Walnuts

50 g Grated coconut

1 teaspoon Cinnamon

Directions:

Roughly chop the dates and soak them in warm water for 15 minutes.

In the meantime, roughly chop the almonds and walnuts.

Drain the dates.

Place the dates with the nuts, coconut and cinnamon in the food processor and mix to an even mass. (But not too long, crispy pieces or nuts make it particularly tasty)

Roll out the mass on 2 baking trays to form an approximately 1 cm thick rectangle.

Cut the rectangle into bars and keep each bar in a piece of parchment paper.

Nutrition:

Calories: 227

Total Fat: 19 g

Sodium: 9 mg

Carbohydrates: 12 g

Protein: 5 g

Hazelnut Balls

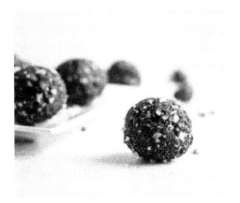

Preparation time: 20 minutes

Cooking time: 4 – 5 hours

Servings: 10

Ingredients:

130 g Dates

140 g Hazelnuts

2 tablespoon Cocoa powder

1 / 2 teaspoon Vanilla extract

1 teaspoon Honey

Directions:

Put the hazelnuts in a food processor and grind them until you get hazelnut flour (you can also use ready-made hazelnut flour).

Put the hazelnut flour in a bowl and set aside.

Put the dates in the food processor and grind them until you get a ball.

Add the hazelnut flour, vanilla extract, cocoa and honey and pulse until you get a nice and even mix.

Remove the mixture from the food processor and turn it into beautiful balls.

Store the balls in the fridge.

Nutrition:

Calories: 73

Total Fat: 5 g

Total Carbohydrates: 5 g

Protein: 1 g

Pine and Sunflower Seed Rolls

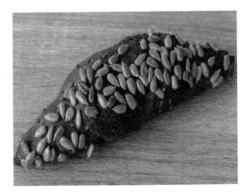

Preparation time: 20 minutes

Cooking time: 35 minutes

Servings: 10

Ingredients:

120 g Tapioca flour

1 teaspoon Celtic sea salt

4 tablespoon Coconut flour

120 ml Olive oil

120 ml Water (warm)

1 piece Egg (beaten)

150 g Pine nuts (roasted)

150 g Sunflower seeds (roasted)

Baking paper sheet

61

Directions:

Preheat the oven to 160 ° C.

Put the pine nuts and sunflower seeds in a small bowl and set aside.

Mix the tapioca with the salt and tablespoons of coconut flour in a large bowl. Pour the olive oil and warm water into the mixture.

Add the egg and mix until you get an even texture. If the dough is too thin, add 1 tablespoon of coconut flour at a time until it has the desired consistency.

Wait a few minutes between each addition of the flour so that it can absorb the moisture. The dough should be soft and sticky.

With a wet tablespoon, take tablespoons of batter to make a roll. Put some tapioca flour on your hands so the dough doesn't stick. Fold the dough with your fingertips instead of rolling it in your palms.

Place the roll in the bowl of pine nuts and sunflower seeds and roll it around until covered.

Line a baking sheet with parchment paper. Place the buns on the baking sheet.

Bake in the preheated oven for 35 minutes and serve warm.

Nutrition:

Calories: 163

Total Fat: 14 g

Fiber: 3 g

Total Carbohydrates: 6.5 g

Protein: 5 g

Banana Dessert

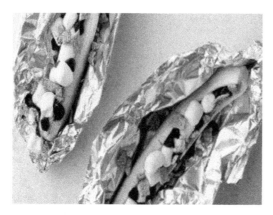

Preparation time: 5 minutes

Cooking time: 4 minutes

Servings: 2

Ingredients:

2 pieces Banana (ripe)

2 tablespoons pure chocolate (70% cocoa)

2 tablespoons Almond leaves

Directions:

Chop the chocolate finely, cut the banana lengthwise, but not completely, as the banana must serve as a casing for the chocolate. Slightly slide on the banana, spread the finely chopped chocolate and almonds over the bananas.

Fold a kind of boat out of the aluminum foil that supports the banana well, with the cut in the banana facing up.

Place the two packets and grill them for about 4 minutes until the skin is dark.

Nutrition:

Calories: 105

Total Fat: 0.4 g

Sodium: 1.2 mg

Total Carbohydrates: 27 g

Protein: 1.3 g

Fiber: 3 g

Strawberry Popsicles with Chocolate Dip

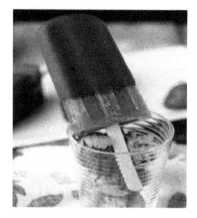

Preparation time: 20 minutes

Cooking time: 5 – 6 hours

Servings: 4

Ingredients:

125 g Strawberries

80 ml Water

100 g pure chocolate (70% cocoa)

Directions:

Clean the strawberries and cut them into pieces. Puree the strawberries with the water.

Pour the mixture into the Popsicle mold and put it in a skewer.

Place the molds in the freezer so the popsicles can freeze hard.

Once the popsicles are frozen hard, you can melt the chocolate in a water bath.

Dip the popsicles in the melted chocolate mixture.

Nutrition:

Calories: 60

Fiber: 1 g

Sugars: 14 g

Total Carbohydrates: 15 g

Strawberry and Coconut Ice Cream

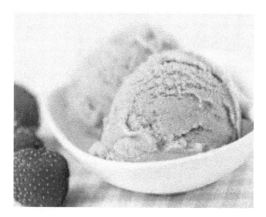

Preparation time: 20 minutes

Cooking time: 1 hour

Servings: 1

Ingredients:

400 ml Coconut milk (can)

1 hand Strawberries

1 / 2 pieces Lime

3 tablespoons Honey

Directions:

Clean the strawberries and cut them into large pieces.

Grate the lime, 1 teaspoon of lime peel is required. Squeeze the lime.

Put all ingredients in a blender and puree everything evenly.

Pour the mixture into a bowl and put it in the freezer for 1 hour.

Take the mixture out of the freezer and put it in the blender. Mix them well again.

Pour the mixture back into the bowl and freeze it until it is hard.

Before serving; take it out of the freezer about 10 minutes before scooping out the balls.

Nutrition:

Calories: 200

Total Fat: 11 g

Cholesterol: 0 mg

Sodium: 5 mg

Total Carbohydrates: 23 g

Protein: 1 g

Coffee Ice Cream

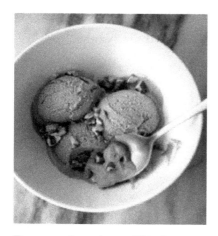

Preparation time: 15 minutes

Cooking time: 1 hour

Servings: 1

Ingredients:

180 ml Coffee

8 pieces Medjool dates

400 ml Coconut milk (can)

1 teaspoon Vanilla extract

Directions:

Make sure that the coffee has cooled down before using it.

Cut the dates into rough pieces.

Place the dates and coffee in a food processor and mix to an even mass.

Add coconut milk and vanilla and puree evenly.

Pour the mixture into a bowl and put it in the freezer for 1 hour.

Take the mixture out of the freezer and scoop it into the blender.

Pour it back into the bowl and freeze it until it's hard.

When serving; take it out of the freezer a few minutes before scooping ice cream balls with a spoon.

Nutrition:

Calories: 140

Total Fat: 7 g

Cholesterol: 25 mg

Sodium: 35 mg

Carbohydrates: 16 g

Banana Strawberry Milkshake

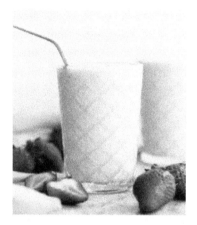

Preparation time: 10 minutes

Cooking time: 10 minutes

Servings: 1

Ingredients:

2 pieces Banana (frozen)

1 hand Strawberries (frozen)

250 ml Coconut milk (can)

Directions:

Peel the bananas, slice them and place them in a bag or on a tray. Put them in the freezer the night before.

Put all ingredients in the blender and mix to an even milkshake.

Spread on the glasses.

Nutrition:

Calories: 110

Total Fat: 1 g

Cholesterol: 5 mg

Sodium: 40 mg

Carbohydrates: 23 g

Sugar: 16 g

Protein: 4 g

Lime and Ginger Green Smoothie

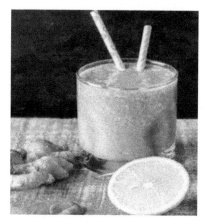

Preparation time: 5 minutes

Cooking time: 5 minutes

Servings: 1

Ingredients:

½ cup dairy free milk

½ cup water

½ teaspoon fresh ginger

½ cup mango chunks

Juice from 1 lime

1 tablespoon dried shredded coconut

1 tablespoon flaxseeds

1 cup spinach

Directions:

Blend together all the ingredients until smooth.

Serve and enjoy!

Nutrition:

Calories 178

Fat 1g

Carbohydrates 7g

Protein 4g

Turmeric Strawberry Green Smoothie

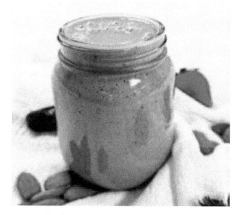

Preparation time: 5 minutes

Cooking time: 5 minutes

Servings: 1

Ingredients:

1 cup kale, stalks removed

1 teaspoon turmeric

1 cup strawberries

½ cup coconut yogurt

6 walnut halves

1 tablespoon raw cacao powder

1-2 mm slice of bird's eye chili

1 cup unsweetened almond milk

1 pitted Medjool date

Directions:

Blend together all the ingredients and enjoy immediately!

Be careful how much almond milk you add so you can choose your favorite consistency.

Nutrition:

Calories 180

Fat 2.2g

Carbohydrates 12g

Protein 4g

Sirtfood Wonder Smoothie

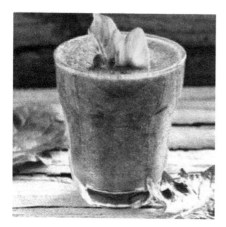

Preparation time: 5 minutes

Cooking time: 10 minutes

Servings: 1

Ingredients:

1 cup arugula (rocket)

2 cups organic strawberries or blueberries

1 cup kale

½ teaspoon matcha green tea

Juice of ½ lemon or lime

3 sprigs of parsley

½ cup of watercress

78

¾ cup of water

Directions:

Add all the ingredients except matcha to a blender and whizz up until very smooth.

Add the matcha green tea powder and give it a final blitz until well mixed.

Nutrition:

Calories 145

Fat 2g

Carbohydrates 7g

Protein 3g

Strawberry Spinach Smoothie

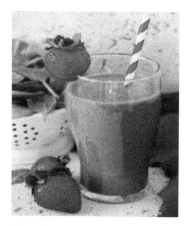

Preparation time: 5 minutes

Cooking time: 5 minutes

Servings: 1

Ingredients:

1 cup whole frozen strawberries

3 cups packed spinach

¼ cup frozen pineapple chunks

1 medium ripe banana, cut into chunks and frozen

1 cup unsweetened milk

1 tablespoon chia seeds

Directions:

Place all the ingredients in a high-powered blender.

Blend until smooth.

Enjoy!

Nutrition:

Calories 266

Fat 8g

Carbohydrates 48g

Protein 9g

Berry Turmeric Smoothie

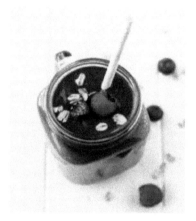

Preparation time: 5 minutes

Cooking time: 5 minutes

Servings: 1

Ingredients:

1 ½ cups frozen mixed berries (blueberries, blackberries and raspberries)

½ teaspoon ground turmeric

2 cups baby spinach

¾ cup unsweetened vanilla almond milk, or milk of choice

½ cup non-fat plain Greek yogurt, or yoghurt of choice

¼ teaspoon ground ginger

2-3 teaspoons honey

3 tablespoons old-fashioned rolled oats

Directions:

Place all the ingredients in a high-powered blender.

Blend until smooth.

Taste and adjust sweetness as desired.

Enjoy immediately!

Nutrition:

Calories 151

Fat 2g

Carbohydrates 27g

Protein 8g

Mango Green Smoothie

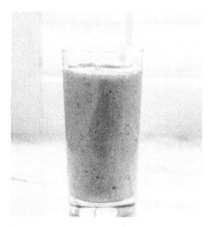

Preparation time: 3 minutes

Cooking time: 5 minutes

Servings: 1

Ingredients:

1 ½ cups frozen mango pieces

1 cup packed baby spinach leaves

1 ripe banana

¾ cup unsweetened vanilla almond milk

Directions:

Place all the ingredients in a blender.

Blend until smooth.

Enjoy!

Nutrition:

Calories 229

Fat 2g

Carbohydrates 72g

Protein 2g

Apple Avocado Smoothie

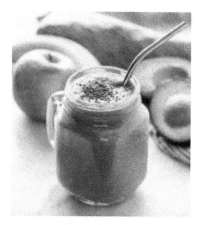

Preparation time: 5 minutes

Cooking time: 5 minutes

Servings: 1

Ingredients:

2 cups packed spinach

½ medium avocados

1 medium apple, peeled and quartered

½ medium bananas, cut into chunks and frozen

½ cup unsweetened almond milk

1 teaspoon honey

¼ teaspoon ground ginger

Small handful of ice cubes

Directions:

In the ordered list, add the almond milk, spinach, avocado, banana, apples, honey, ginger, and ice to a high-powered blender.

Blend until smooth.

Taste and adjust sweetness and spices as desired.

Enjoy immediately!

Nutrition:

Calories 206

Fat 11g

Carbohydrates 15g

Protein 5g

Kale Pineapple Smoothie

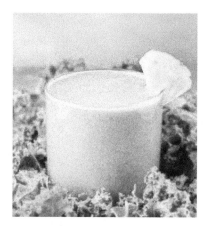

Preparation time: 5 minutes

Cooking time: 5 minutes

Servings: 1

Ingredients:

2 cups lightly packed chopped kale leaves, stems removed

¼ cup frozen pineapple pieces

1 frozen medium banana, cut into chunks

¼ cup non-fat Greek yogurt

2 teaspoons honey

¾ cup unsweetened vanilla almond milk, or any milk of choice

2 tablespoons peanut butter, creamy or crunchy

Directions:

Place all the ingredients in a blender.

Blend until smooth.

Add more milk as needed to reach desired consistency.

Enjoy immediately!

Nutrition:

Calories 187

Fat 9g

Carbohydrates 27g

Protein 8g

Blueberry Banana Avocado Smoothie

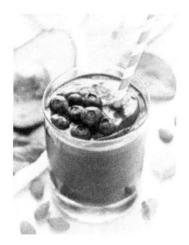

Preparation time: 10 minutes

Cooking time: 10 minutes

Servings: 1

Ingredients:

1 medium ripe banana, peeled

2 cups frozen blueberries

1 cup fresh spinach

1 tablespoon ground flaxseed meal

½ ripe avocados

1 tablespoon almond butter

¼ teaspoon cinnamon

½ cup unsweetened vanilla almond milk

Directions:

Place all the ingredients in your blender in the ordered list: vanilla almond milk, spinach, banana, avocado, blueberries, flaxseed meal, and almond butter.

Blend until smooth.

If you like a thicker smoothie, add a small handful of ice.

Enjoy immediately!

Nutrition:

Calories 298

Fat 14.4g

Carbohydrates 38.1g

Protein 8g

Carrot Smoothie

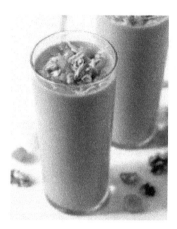

Preparation time: 10 minutes

Cooking time: 10 minutes

Servings: 1

Ingredients:

1 cup chopped carrots

¼ cup frozen diced pineapple

½ cup frozen sliced banana

¼ teaspoon cinnamon

1 tablespoon flaked coconut

½ cup Greek yogurt

2 tablespoons toasted walnuts

Pinch nutmeg

½ cup unsweetened vanilla almond milk, or milk of choice

For topping:

Shredded carrots, coconut, crushed walnuts

Directions:

Add all the ingredients into a blender.

Blend until smooth.

Enjoy immediately, topped with additional shredded carrots, coconut, and crushed walnuts as desired!

Nutrition:

Calories 279

Fat 6g

Carbohydrates 48g

Protein 7g

Matcha Berry Smoothie

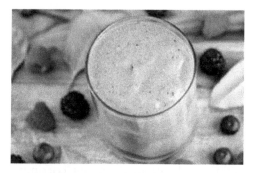

Preparation time: 5 minutes

Cooking time: 5 minutes

Servings: 1

Ingredients:

½ bananas

½-tablespoon matcha powder

1 cup almond milk

1 cup frozen blueberries

¼ teaspoon ground ginger

½ tablespoon chia seeds

¼ teaspoon ground cinnamon

Directions:

In a blender, blend the almond milk, banana, blueberries, matcha powder, chia seeds, cinnamon, and ginger until smooth.

Enjoy immediately!

Nutrition:

Calories 212

Fat 5g

Carbohydrates 34g

Protein 8g

Simple Grape Smoothie

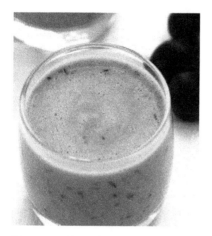

Preparation time: 5 minutes

Cooking time: 5 minutes

Servings: 1

Ingredients:

2 cups red seedless grapes

¼ cup grape juice

½ cup plain yogurt

1 cup ice

Directions:

Add grape juice to the blender. Then add yogurt and grapes. Add the ice last.

Blend until smooth and enjoy!

Nutrition:

Calories 161

Fat 4g

Carbohydrates 39g

Protein 2g

Ginger Plum Smoothie

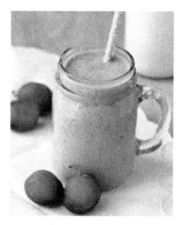

Preparation time: 5 minutes

Cooking time: 5 minutes

Servings: 1

Ingredients:

1 ripe plum, fresh or frozen, pitted but not peeled

½ cup plain yogurt

½ cup orange juice, or other fruit juice

1 teaspoon grated fresh ginger

Directions:

Put all the ingredients in a blender and blend until smooth.

Serve immediately and enjoy!

Nutrition:

Calories 124

Fat 2g

Carbohydrates 26g

Protein 3g

Kumquat Mango Smoothie

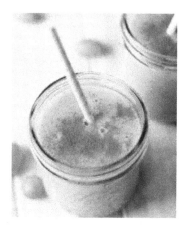

Preparation time: 10 minutes

Cooking time: 5 minutes

Servings: 1

Ingredients:

15 small kumquats

½ mango, peeled and chopped

¾ cup unsweetened almond milk

¼ teaspoon vanilla

½ cup plain yogurt

¼ teaspoon nutmeg

1 tablespoon honey

100

½ teaspoon ground cinnamon

5 ice cubes

Directions:

Cut the kumquats in half and remove any seeds.

Add all the ingredients to a blender and blend until smooth.

Garnish with another sprinkling of cinnamon, if desired.

Enjoy immediately!

Nutrition:

Calories 116

Fat 2g

Carbohydrates 22g

Protein 5g

Cranberry Smoothie

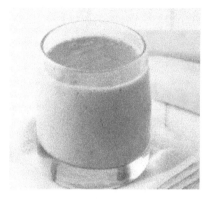

Preparation time: 5 minutes

Cooking time: 5 minutes

Servings: 1

Ingredients:

½ cup frozen cranberries

½ bananas

¼ cup orange juice

¼ cup frozen blueberries

¼ cup low fat Greek yogurt

Directions:

Add all the ingredients to a blender and blend until smooth.

Add a little more orange juice if you prefer it a little thinner. Enjoy immediately!

Nutrition:

Calories 165

Fat 1g

Carbohydrates 31g

Protein 8g

Summer Berry Smoothie

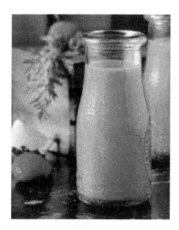

Preparation time: 10 minutes

Cooking time: 10 minutes

Servings: 1

Ingredients:

50g (2oz) blueberries

50g (2oz) strawberries

25g (1oz) blackcurrants

25g (1oz) red grapes

1 carrot, peeled

1 orange, peeled

Juice of 1 lime

Directions:

Place all of the ingredients into a blender and cover them with water.

Blitz until smooth.

You can also add some crushed ice and a mint leaf to garnish.

Nutrition:

Calories: 110

Fat: 1 g

Carbohydrates: 20 g

Protein: 2 g

Mango, Celery and Ginger Smoothie

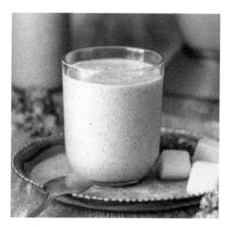

Preparation time: 10 minutes

Cooking time: 10 minutes

Servings: 1

Ingredients:

1 stalk of celery

50g (2oz) kale

1 apple, cored

50g (2oz) mango, peeled, de-stoned and chopped

2.5cm (1 inch) chunk of fresh ginger root, peeled and chopped

Directions:

Put all the ingredients into a blender with some water and blitz until smooth. Add ice to make your smoothie really refreshing.

Nutrition:

Calories: 92

Fat: 3 g

Carbohydrates: 22 g

Protein: 1 g

Orange, Carrot and Kale Smoothie

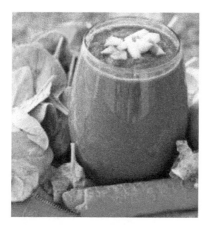

Preparation time: 5 minutes

Cooking time: 5 minutes

Servings: 1

Ingredients:

1 carrot, peeled

1 orange, peeled

1 stick of celery

1 apple, cored

50g (2oz) kale

½ teaspoon matcha powder

Directions:

Place all of the ingredients into a blender and add in enough water to cover them. Process until smooth, serve and enjoy.

Nutrition:

Calories: 150

Fat: 1 g

Carbohydrates: 36 g

Protein: 4 g

Creamy Strawberry and Cherry Smoothie

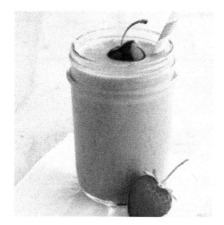

Preparation time: 5 minutes

Cooking time: 5 minutes

Servings: 1

Ingredients:

100g (3½ oz) strawberries

75g (3oz) frozen pitted cherries

1 tablespoon plain full-fat yogurt

175mls (6fl oz) unsweetened soya milk

Directions:

Place all of the ingredients into a blender and process until smooth.

Serve and enjoy.

Nutrition:

Calories: 135

Fat: 1 g

Carbohydrates: 25 g

Protein: 3 g

Pineapple and Cucumber Smoothie

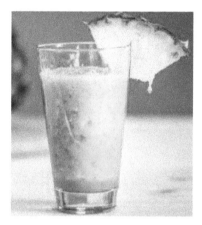

Preparation time: 5 minutes

Cooking time: 5 minutes

Servings: 1

Ingredients:

50g (2oz) cucumber

1 stalk of celery

2 slices of fresh pineapple

2 sprigs of parsley

½ teaspoon matcha powder

Squeeze of lemon juice

Directions:

Place all of the ingredients into blender with enough water to cover them and blitz until smooth.

Nutrition:

Calories: 125

Fat: 1 g

Carbohydrates: 22 g

Protein: 2 g

Avocado, Celery and Pineapple Smoothie

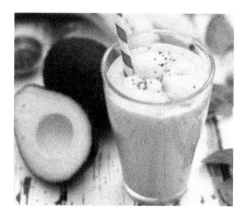

Preparation time: 5 minutes

Cooking time: 5 minutes

Servings: 1

Ingredients:

50g (2oz) fresh pineapple, peeled and chopped

3 stalks of celery

1 avocado, peeled & de-stoned

1 teaspoon fresh parsley

½ teaspoon matcha powder

Juice of ½ lemons

Directions:

Place all of the ingredients into a blender and add enough water to cover them - process until creamy and smooth.

Nutrition:

Calories: 138

Fat: 2 g

Carbohydrates: 25 g

Protein: 5g

Mango and Rocket (Arugula) Smoothie

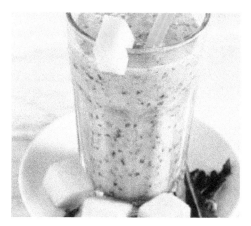

Preparation time: 5 minutes

Cooking time: 5 minutes

Servings: 1

Ingredients:

25g (1oz) fresh rocket (arugula)

150g (5oz) fresh mango, peeled, de-stoned and chopped

1 avocado, de-stoned and peeled

½ teaspoon matcha powder

Juice of 1 lime

Directions:

Place all of the ingredients into a blender with enough water to cover them and process until smooth. Add a few ice cubes and enjoy.

Nutrition:

Calories: 145

Fat: 2 g

Carbohydrates: 21 g

Protein: 5 g

Strawberry and Citrus Blend

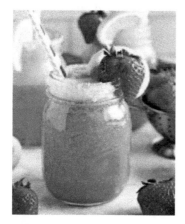

Preparation time: 5 minutes

Cooking time: 5 minutes

Servings: 1

Ingredients:

75g (3oz) strawberries

1 apple, cored

1 orange, peeled

½ avocado, peeled and de-stoned

½ teaspoon matcha powder

Juice of 1 lime

Directions:

Place all of the ingredients into a blender with enough water to cover them and process until smooth. Add ice to make it really refreshing.

Nutrition:

Calories: 112

Fat: 2 g

Carbohydrates: 23 g

Protein: 1 g

Orange and Celery Crush

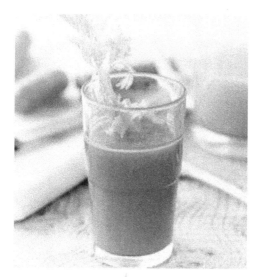

Preparation time: 5 minutes

Cooking time: 5 minutes

Servings: 1

Ingredients:

1 carrot, peeled

3 stalks of celery

1 orange, peeled

½ teaspoon matcha powder

Juice of 1 lime

Directions:

Place all of the ingredients into a blender with enough water to cover them and blitz until smooth. Add crushed ice to make your smoothie really refreshing.

Nutrition:

Calories: 180

Fat: 2 g

Carbohydrates: 25 g

Protein: 3 g

Chocolate, Strawberry and Coconut Crush

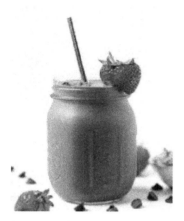

Preparation time: 5 minutes

Cooking time: 5 minutes

Servings: 1

Ingredients:

100mls (3½fl oz) coconut milk

100g (3½oz) strawberries

1 banana

1 tablespoon 100% cocoa powder or cacao nibs

1 teaspoon matcha powder

Directions:

Toss all of the ingredients into a blender and process them to a creamy consistency.

Add a little extra water if you need to thin it a little. Add crushed ice to make your smoothie really refreshing.

Nutrition:

Calories: 220

Fat: 3 g

Carbohydrates: 30 g

Protein: 5 g

Banana and Kale Smoothie

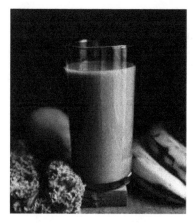

Preparation time: 5 minutes

Cooking time: 5 minutes

Servings: 1

Ingredients:

50g (2oz) kale

1 banana

200mls (7fl oz) unsweetened soya milk

Directions:

Place all of the ingredients into a blender with enough water to cover them and process until smooth. Add ice to make it really refreshing.

Nutrition:

Calories: 189

Fat: 2 g

Carbohydrates: 25 g

Protein: 3 g

Cranberry and Kale Crush

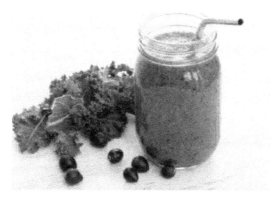

Preparation time: 5 minutes

Cooking time: 5 minutes

Servings: 1

Ingredients:

75g (3oz) strawberries

50g (2oz) kale

120mls (4fl oz) unsweetened cranberry juice

1 teaspoon chia seeds

½ teaspoon matcha powder

Directions:

Place all of the ingredients into a blender and process until smooth. Add some crushed ice and a mint leaf or two for a really refreshing drink.

Nutrition:

Calories: 213

Fat: 1 g

Carbohydrates: 28 g

Protein: 3 g

Grape, Celery and Parsley Reviver

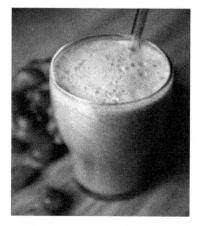

Preparation time: 5 minutes

Cooking time: 5 minutes

Servings: 1

Ingredients:

75g (3oz) red grapes

3 sticks of celery

1 avocado, de-stoned and peeled

1 tablespoon fresh parsley

½ teaspoon matcha powder

Directions:

Place all of the ingredients into a blender with enough water to cover them and blitz until smooth and creamy. Add crushed ice to make it even more refreshing.

Nutrition:

Calories: 253

Fat: 2 g

Carbohydrates: 35 g

Protein: 3 g

Grapefruit and Celery Blast

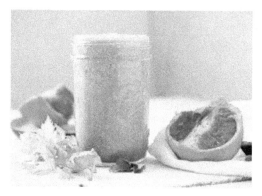

Preparation time: 5 minutes

Cooking time: 5 minutes

Servings: 1

Ingredients:

1 grapefruit, peeled

2 stalks of celery

50g (2oz) kale

½ teaspoon matcha powder

Directions:

Place all the ingredients into a blender with enough water to cover them and blitz until smooth.

Add crushed ice to make it even more refreshing.

Nutrition:

Calories: 220

Fat: 1 g

Carbohydrates: 31 g

Protein: 2 g

Tropical Chocolate Delight

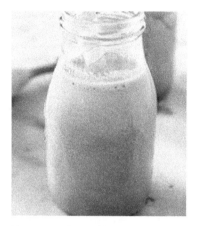

Preparation time: 5 minutes

Cooking time: 5 minutes

Servings: 1

Ingredients:

1 mango, peeled & de-stoned

75g (3oz) fresh pineapple, chopped

50g (2oz) kale

25g (1oz) rocket

1 tablespoon 100% cocoa powder or cacao nibs

150mls (5fl oz) coconut milk

Directions:

Place all of the ingredients into a blender and blitz until smooth. You can add a little water if it seems too thick.

Add crushed ice to make it even more refreshing.

Nutrition:

Calories: 289

Fat: 4 g

Carbohydrates: 37 g

Protein: 3 g

CPSIA information can be obtained
at www.ICGtesting.com
Printed in the USA
BVHW091109230221
600894BV00002B/231